I0696907

Watch Your Weight New Complete Cookbook.

Delectable Recipes for a Healthy and Nutritious Kitchen.

By Priscilla Clayton.

Copyright.

Table of Contents.

Soups

- Chicken taco soup
- Buffalo chicken soup. etc

Snacks

- Turkey sausage rolls
- Onion cheese rings. etc

International Flavors

Vegetable Upma (Indian Semolina Breakfast).

Japanese Tamago Sando (Egg Salad Sandwich).

Etc

Understanding Weight Watchers.

Weight Watchers, now known as WW, is a popular and well-established weight loss and wellness program. Founded in the 1960s, its approach has evolved over the years, focusing on helping individuals make healthier food choices and adopt a more active lifestyle. The core principle of Weight Watchers is to assign a point value to different foods based on their nutritional content. Participants are given a daily points target to stay within, encouraging them to make balanced and mindful food choices.

The program also emphasizes community support as a vital component of success. Members attend group meetings or engage in online communities to share their experiences, challenges, and achievements. In recent years, WW has incorporated technology, offering a mobile app that assists users in tracking their food intake, physical activity, and progress toward their goals.

The flexibility of the program allows individuals to choose the foods they enjoy while still adhering to their point target. This approach promotes a sustainable lifestyle change rather than a temporary diet. WW has also expanded its focus beyond weight loss to encompass overall well-being, including mental health, mindful eating, and self-care.

Kitchen Essentials for Healthy Cooking.

Creating nutritious and delicious meals starts with having the right tools in your kitchen. Here are some essential items for healthy cooking:

Quality Cookware: Invest in non-stick pans, stainless steel pots, and baking sheets to minimize the need for excessive cooking oils.

Sharp Knives: A set of sharp knives makes chopping vegetables and preparing ingredients easier and safer.

Cutting Boards: Opt for durable, easy-to-clean cutting boards. Having separate boards for raw meats and produce helps prevent cross-contamination.

Steamer Basket: Steaming vegetables helps retain their nutrients and natural flavors. A steamer basket is a versatile tool for quick and healthy cooking.

Blender or Food Processor: These appliances are perfect for making smoothies, soups, and homemade sauces using fresh ingredients.

Measuring Tools: Accurate portion control is crucial for maintaining a balanced diet. Measuring cups and spoons help you keep track of serving sizes.

Grill Pan or Outdoor Grill: Grilling is a healthier cooking method that imparts a unique flavor to foods. Consider a grill pan for indoor use or an outdoor grill for barbecues.

Herbs and Spices: Build a collection of herbs and spices to add flavor to your dishes without relying on excessive salt, sugar, or fats.

Non-Stick Cooking Spray: A light spritz of cooking spray can help reduce the amount of oil needed when sautéing or baking.

Storage Containers: Having a variety of storage containers on hand makes it easy to pack leftovers for healthy lunches or meal prep.

Salad Spinner: Washing and drying leafy greens becomes a breeze with a salad spinner, promoting the consumption of fresh salads.

Oven Thermometer: Ensure your oven is at the correct temperature for baking and roasting, ensuring consistent and perfectly cooked meals.

Breakfast Ideas.

A). Healthy Morning Starts.

1. Fluffy Whole Wheat Pancakes.

Ingredients:

- 1 cup whole wheat flour
- 1 tablespoon sugar
- 1 teaspoon baking powder
- 1/2 teaspoon baking soda
- 1/4 teaspoon salt
- 1 cup buttermilk
- 1/4 cup milk
- 1 egg

- 2 tablespoons melted butter

Directions:

1. In a mixing bowl, whisk together the whole wheat flour, sugar, baking powder, baking soda, and salt.
2. In another bowl, whisk together the buttermilk, milk, egg, and melted butter until well combined.
3. Pour the wet ingredients into the dry ingredients and gently mix until just combined. Be careful not to overmix; a few lumps are okay.
4. Heat a non-stick skillet or griddle over medium heat.
5. Grease lightly with butter or cooking spray.

6. Pour about 1/4 cup of batter onto the skillet for each pancake.

7. Cook until bubbles form on the surface, then flip and cook until the other side is golden brown.

8. Serve the fluffy whole wheat pancakes with your favorite toppings, such as fresh fruit, maple syrup, or yogurt.

Nutrition Information (per serving):

- Calories: 150
- Carbohydrates: 22g
- Protein: 5g
- Fat: 4g
- Fiber: 3g

<u>2. Scrambled Egg Whites with Spinach and Tomatoes.</u>

Ingredients:

- 4 egg whites
- 1 cup fresh spinach, chopped
- 1/2 cup cherry tomatoes, halved
- Salt and pepper to taste
- 1 teaspoon olive oil

Directions:

1. Heat the olive oil in a non-stick skillet over medium heat.
2. Add the cherry tomatoes and sauté for a few minutes until they start to soften.
3. Add the chopped spinach to the skillet and cook until wilted.

4. Push the tomatoes and spinach to one side of the skillet and pour in the egg whites.

5. Let the egg whites sit for a moment, then gently scramble them with a spatula as they begin to set.

6. Continue cooking and scrambling until the egg whites are fully cooked and fluffy.

7. Season with salt and pepper to taste.

8. Serve the scrambled egg whites with spinach and tomatoes as a healthy and protein-packed breakfast option.

Nutrition Information (per serving):

- Calories: 100
- Carbohydrates: 6g
- Protein: 15g
- Fat: 2g
- Fiber: 2g

Ingredients:

- Assorted fresh fruits (e.g., strawberries, blueberries, kiwi, pineapple, grapes, etc.)
- 1 cup plain yogurt
- 1 tablespoon honey
- 1 teaspoon vanilla extract (optional)

Directions:

1. Wash, peel, and chop the fresh fruits into bite-sized pieces.
2. In a bowl, mix the plain yogurt, honey, and vanilla extract (if using) until well combined.

3. Gently fold the chopped fruits into the yogurt mixture, ensuring they are evenly coated.

4. Refrigerate the fruit salad for at least 30 minutes to allow the flavors to meld.

5. Serve the fresh fruit salad with a dollop of additional yogurt on top if desired.

Nutrition Information.

- Calories: 150 (varies based on fruit used)
- Carbohydrates: 30g
- Protein: 5g
- Fat: 2g
- Fiber: 4g

4. Instant Pot Egg Bites.

<u>*Ingredients:*</u>

- 4 large eggs
- 1/2 cup cottage cheese
- 1/4 cup shredded cheddar cheese
- 1/4 cup cooked and crumbled bacon or diced ham
- 1/4 cup diced bell peppers
- Salt and pepper to taste

<u>*Directions:*</u>

1. In a blender, combine the eggs, cottage cheese, and shredded cheddar cheese. Blend until smooth.
2. Stir in the cooked bacon or ham and diced bell peppers.

3. Season with salt and pepper.

4. Grease the egg bite molds or silicone molds with non-stick cooking spray.

5. Pour the egg mixture evenly into the molds, filling each about 3/4 full.

6. Add 1 cup of water to the Instant Pot. Place the trivet inside.

7. Carefully place the molds on the trivet.

8. Close the Instant Pot lid and set the valve to the sealing position.

9. Cook on high pressure for 8-10 minutes.

10. Once done, allow natural pressure release for 5 minutes, then do a quick release.

11. Carefully remove the molds from the Instant Pot and let the egg bites cool slightly before serving.

Nutrition Information (per serving):

- Calories: ~120
- Protein: ~10g
- Carbohydrates: ~2g
- Fat: ~8g
- Fiber: ~0.2g

5. Tater Tot Breakfast Casserole.

Ingredients:

- 2 cups frozen tater tots
- 1 cup cooked breakfast sausage
- 1 cup shredded cheddar cheese
- 6 large eggs
- 1/2 cup milk
- Salt and pepper to taste
- Chopped green onions for garnish

1. Preheat the oven to 375°F (190°C) and grease a baking dish.
2. Spread the frozen tater tots in an even layer in the baking dish.
3. Sprinkle the cooked breakfast sausage and shredded cheddar cheese over the tater tots.
4. In a bowl, whisk together the eggs, milk, salt, and pepper.
5. Pour the egg mixture over the tater tot mixture.
6. Bake in the preheated oven for 25-30 minutes, or until the eggs are set and the top is golden.
7. Remove from the oven and let it cool slightly before serving.

8. Garnish with chopped green onions before serving.

Nutrition Information (per serving):

- Calories: ~350
- Protein: ~18g
- Carbohydrates: ~20g
- Fat: ~22g
- Fiber: ~1g

6. Turkey Breakfast Sausage Patties.

Ingredients:

- 1 pound ground turkey
- 1 teaspoon ground sage

- 1/2 teaspoon dried thyme
- 1/2 teaspoon garlic powder
- 1/2 teaspoon onion powder
- 1/4 teaspoon crushed red pepper flakes (optional)
- Salt and pepper to taste

Directions:

1. In a mixing bowl, combine the ground turkey, ground sage, dried thyme, garlic powder, onion powder, crushed red pepper flakes (if using), salt, and pepper.
2. Mix the ingredients until well combined.
3. Divide the mixture into equal portions and shape them into patties.
4. Heat a non-stick skillet over medium heat.
5. Place the turkey patties in the skillet and cook for about 3-4 minutes on each side,

or until they are cooked through and no longer pink in the center.

6. Remove the patties from the skillet and drain on paper towels.

Nutrition Information .

- Calories: 150
- Protein: 20g
- Fat: 7g
- Carbohydrates: 1g
- Fiber: 0g

7. Breakfast Taco Bowl.

Ingredients:

- 2 large eggs

- 1/2 cup black beans, drained and rinsed
- 1/4 cup diced tomatoes
- 1/4 cup diced bell peppers
- 2 tablespoons diced red onion
- 1/4 avocado, sliced
- 1 tablespoon chopped fresh cilantro
- Salt and pepper to taste
- 1 tablespoon olive oil
- 1 small corn tortilla, baked until crispy (optional)

<u>Directions:</u>

1. Heat olive oil in a skillet over medium heat.
2. Add diced tomatoes, bell peppers, and red onion to the skillet. Sauté for a few minutes until vegetables are slightly softened.

3. Push the vegetables to the side and crack the eggs into the skillet. Scramble them until cooked to your preference.

4. Add black beans to the skillet and stir to heat them.

5. Season with salt and pepper.

6. In a bowl, assemble the cooked mixture, sliced avocado, and chopped cilantro.

7. Serve with a crispy corn tortilla if desired.

Nutrition Information;

- Calories: 280
- Protein: 14g
- Fat: 18g
- Carbohydrates: 16g
- Fiber: 7g

8. Banana Blueberry Muffins.

<u>*Ingredients:*</u>

- 2 ripe bananas, mashed
- 1/4 cup honey or maple syrup
- 1/4 cup unsweetened applesauce
- 1 large egg
- 1 teaspoon vanilla extract
- 1 cup whole wheat flour
- 1 teaspoon baking powder
- 1/2 teaspoon baking soda
- 1/2 teaspoon ground cinnamon
- Pinch of salt
- 1/2 cup fresh or frozen blueberries

<u>*Directions:*</u>

1. Preheat the oven to 350°F (175°C) and line a muffin tin with paper liners.

2. In a bowl, mix the mashed bananas, honey or maple syrup, applesauce, egg, and vanilla extract until well combined.

3. In a separate bowl, whisk together the whole wheat flour, baking powder, baking soda, ground cinnamon, and salt.

4. Gradually add the dry ingredients to the wet ingredients and stir until just combined.

5. Gently fold in the blueberries.

6. Divide the batter evenly among the muffin cups, filling each about 3/4 full.

7. Bake for 18-20 minutes, or until a toothpick inserted into the center of a muffin comes out clean.

8. Allow the muffins to cool in the tin for a few minutes before transferring to a wire rack to cool completely.

Nutrition Information:

- Calories: 120
- Protein: 2g
- Fat: 1g
- Carbohydrates: 28g
- Fiber: 3g

B).Energizing Oat .

9. Classic Oatmeal with Berries and Nuts.

Ingredients:

- 1 cup rolled oats

- 2 cups milk (or water for a lighter option)

- Pinch of salt

- 1/2 cup mixed berries (strawberries, blueberries, raspberries)

- 1/4 cup chopped nuts (almonds, walnuts, or your choice)

- Honey or maple syrup for sweetening (optional)

Directions:

1. In a saucepan, bring the milk (or water) to a gentle boil.

2. Stir in the rolled oats and a pinch of salt. Reduce heat to medium-low.

3. Cook the oats, stirring occasionally, for about 5-7 minutes or until they reach your desired consistency.

4. Remove from heat and let the oatmeal sit for a minute before serving.

5. Top with mixed berries, chopped nuts, and a drizzle of honey or maple syrup if desired.

10. Overnight Chia Seed Oats.

Ingredients:

- 1/2 cup rolled oats
- 2 tbsp chia seeds
- 1/2 cup yogurt (or milk of choice)

- 1/2 cup chopped fruits (banana, mango, etc.)
- 1 tsp honey or sweetener of choice (optional)

Directions:

1. In a jar or container, combine the rolled oats, chia seeds, and yogurt (or milk).
2. Stir well, ensuring that the oats and chia seeds are fully submerged.
3. Cover and refrigerate overnight or for at least 4 hours.
4. Before serving, give the mixture a good stir and top with chopped fruits and a drizzle of honey or sweetener.

11. Savory Oat and Vegetable Muffins.

<u>*Ingredients:*</u>

- 1 cup rolled oats
- 1 cup whole wheat flour
- 1 tsp baking powder
- 1/2 tsp baking soda
- Salt and pepper to taste
- 1 cup buttermilk or yogurt
- 1 egg
- 1/4 cup melted butter or oil
- 1 cup chopped mixed vegetables (spinach, bell peppers, onions, etc.)
- 1/2 cup grated cheese (cheddar, mozzarella, etc.)

<u>*Directions:*</u>

1. Preheat the oven to 350°F (175°C) and grease a muffin tin.

2. In a bowl, mix the oats, whole wheat flour, baking powder, baking soda, salt, and pepper.

3. In another bowl, whisk together the buttermilk or yogurt, egg, and melted butter or oil.

4. Combine the wet and dry ingredients, then fold in the chopped vegetables and grated cheese.

5. Spoon the mixture into the muffin tin, filling each cup about 3/4 full.

6. Bake for 20-25 minutes or until the muffins are golden brown and a toothpick inserted into the center comes out clean.

<u>**C). Protein-Packed Choices**</u>

<u>**12. Greek Yogurt Parfait with Granola and Honey.**</u>

Ingredients:

- Greek yogurt
- Granola
- Honey
- Fresh fruits (e.g., berries, bananas)

Directions:

1. In a glass or bowl, start by adding a layer of Greek yogurt.
2. Sprinkle a layer of granola on top of the yogurt.

3. Add a drizzle of honey over the granola.

4. Add a layer of fresh fruits.

5. Repeat the layers until you achieve your desired portion.

6. Enjoy immediately or refrigerate until ready to eat.

13. Quinoa and Veggie Breakfast Bowl.

Ingredients:

- Quinoa
- Assorted vegetables (e.g., spinach, bell peppers, tomatoes, onions)
- Eggs
- Olive oil
- Salt and pepper

- Optional: avocado, feta cheese, herbs

Directions:

1. Rinse quinoa thoroughly and cook according to package instructions.
2. While quinoa is cooking, chop vegetables.
3. In a pan, heat olive oil and sauté vegetables until they're tender.
4. Push the vegetables to the side of the pan and crack eggs into the other side.
5. Scramble the eggs and mix them with the cooked vegetables.
6. Season with salt and pepper.
7. In a bowl, place a serving of cooked quinoa.
8. Top with the egg and vegetable mixture.
9. Add optional toppings like avocado slices, crumbled feta cheese, and herbs.

10.Mix well before eating.

Nutrition Information.

- Quinoa is a complete protein and provides dietary fiber.
- Vegetables offer vitamins, minerals, and antioxidants.
- Eggs contribute additional protein and nutrients.
- Olive oil provides healthy fats.

14. Turkey Sausage and Egg Breakfast Burrito.

Ingredients:

- Whole wheat tortilla

- Cooked turkey sausage

- Eggs

- Bell peppers

- Onions

- Spinach

- Cheese (optional)

- Salt and pepper

Directions:

1. In a pan, cook turkey sausage until browned and fully cooked. Set aside.

2. In the same pan, sauté chopped bell peppers and onions until they're tender.

3. Add spinach and cook until wilted.

4. Beat eggs, season with salt and pepper, and scramble in the pan with the vegetables.

5. Warm the whole wheat tortilla in a dry pan or microwave.

6. Place the scrambled egg and vegetable mixture onto the tortilla.

7. Add cooked turkey sausage on top.

8. If desired, sprinkle cheese over the mixture.

9. Roll up the tortilla, folding in the sides to make a burrito.

D). Creative Toast Variations.

15. Avocado and Poached Egg Toast.

Ingredients:

- 1 ripe avocado

- 2 eggs

- 2 slices of whole-grain bread

- Salt and pepper, to taste

- Optional toppings: red pepper flakes, chopped fresh herbs

Directions:

1. Cut the avocado in half, remove the pit, and scoop the flesh into a bowl. Mash the avocado with a fork and season with salt and pepper.

2. Toast the slices of whole-grain bread until they are golden and crispy.

3. While the bread is toasting, poach the eggs. Bring a pot of water to a gentle simmer and add a splash of vinegar.

4. Crack each egg into a small bowl, then gently slide them into the simmering

41

water. Poach for about 3-4 minutes for a soft, runny yolk.

5. Carefully remove the poached eggs with a slotted spoon and place them on a paper towel to drain any excess water.

6. Spread the mashed avocado evenly onto the toasted bread slices.

7. Place a poached egg on top of each slice of bread.

8. Add optional toppings like red pepper flakes or chopped fresh herbs for extra flavor.

9. Season with additional salt and pepper if desired.

Nutrition Information

- Calories: 350-400 per serving
- Protein: 15-20g

- Carbohydrates: 25-30g

- Dietary Fiber: 10-15g

- Healthy Fats: 20-25g

- Vitamins and Minerals: Rich in vitamin E, vitamin K, potassium, and folate.

16. Almond Butter and Banana Toast.

Ingredients:

- L

- 2 tablespoons almond butter

- 1 banana, sliced

- 2 slices of whole-grain bread

- Honey or cinnamon (optional)

Directions:

1. Toast the slices of whole-grain bread until they are golden and crispy.

2. Spread a tablespoon of almond butter onto each slice of toasted bread.

3. Arrange the banana slices on top of the almond butter.

4. Drizzle with honey or sprinkle with cinnamon if desired.

Nutrition Information.

- Calories: 300-350 per serving
- Protein: 8-10g
- Carbohydrates: 40-45g
- Dietary Fiber: 7-9g
- Healthy Fats: 14-16g
- Vitamins and Minerals: Good source of vitamin E, potassium, and magnesium.

<u>17. Cottage Cheese and Tomato Toast.</u>

<u>Ingredients:</u>

- 1/2 cup low-fat cottage cheese
- 1 large tomato, sliced
- 2 slices of whole-grain bread
- Fresh basil leaves, chopped
- Balsamic vinegar (optional)

<u>Directions:</u>

1. Toast the slices of whole-grain bread until they are golden and crispy.
2. Spread a generous layer of low-fat cottage cheese onto each slice of toasted bread.
3. Place the sliced tomatoes on top of the cottage cheese.

4. Sprinkle chopped fresh basil leaves over the tomatoes.

5. Drizzle with balsamic vinegar if desired.

Nutrition Information

- Calories: 250-300 per serving
- Protein: 15-20g
- Carbohydrates: 30-35g
- Dietary Fiber: 6-8g
- Healthy Fats: 5-7g
- Vitamins and Minerals: Excellent source of calcium, vitamin C, and potassium.

E). Smoothies and Shakes

Ingredients:

- 1 cup kale leaves (stems removed)
- 1 cup pineapple chunks (fresh or frozen)
- 1 banana
- 1/2 cup Greek yogurt
- 1/2 cup almond milk (or any milk of your choice)
- 1 tablespoon chia seeds
- Honey or maple syrup (optional, for sweetness)
- Ice cubes

Directions:

1. Wash and chop the kale leaves into manageable pieces.
2. In a blender, combine the kale, pineapple chunks, banana, Greek yogurt, almond milk, and chia seeds.
3. If desired, add a drizzle of honey or maple syrup for sweetness.
4. Blend until the mixture is smooth and creamy.
5. Add ice cubes and blend again until the smoothie reaches your desired consistency.
6. Pour into glasses and enjoy immediately.

Nutrition Information:

- Calories: Approximately 220
- Protein: 8g
- Fiber: 6g

19. Berry Blast Protein Shake.

Ingredients:

- 1 cup mixed berries (strawberries, blueberries, raspberries)
- 1 scoop of your favorite protein powder (whey, plant-based, etc.)
- 1/2 cup Greek yogurt
- 1/2 cup almond milk (or any milk of your choice)
- 1 tablespoon flaxseeds
- 1 teaspoon honey or agave syrup (optional)
- Ice cubes

Directions:

1. Wash the berries and remove any stems.
2. In a blender, combine the mixed berries, protein powder, Greek yogurt, almond milk, flaxseeds, and honey/agave syrup (if using).
3. Blend until the mixture is smooth and well combined.
4. Add ice cubes and blend again until the shake is thick and creamy.
5. Pour into a glass and enjoy immediately.

Nutrition Information:

- Calories: Approximately 250
- Protein: 25g (varies based on protein powder)
- Fiber: 8g

<u>20. Chocolate Banana Protein Smoothie.</u>

<u>Ingredients:</u>

- 1 banana
- 1 scoop chocolate protein powder
- 1 tablespoon cocoa powder
- 1 tablespoon peanut butter
- 1 cup milk (dairy or non-dairy)
- Ice cubes

<u>Directions:</u>

1. Peel the banana and break it into chunks.

2. In a blender, combine the banana chunks, chocolate protein powder, cocoa powder, peanut butter, and milk.

3. Blend until the mixture is creamy and all ingredients are well mixed.

4. Add ice cubes and blend again until the smoothie is thick and frothy.

5. Pour into a glass and enjoy immediately.

Nutrition Information:

- Calories: Approximately 350
- Protein: Approximately 20g (varies based on protein powder)
- Fiber: 5g

Launch Ideas.

21. Chicken Burrito Bowl.

Ingredients:

- Cooked chicken breast, shredded
- Cooked rice (white or brown)
- Black beans, drained and rinsed
- Corn kernels
- Chopped lettuce
- Diced tomatoes
- Sliced avocado
- Shredded cheese (cheddar or Mexican blend)
- Sour cream

- Salsa or pico de gallo

- Lime wedges

- Fresh cilantro (optional)

<u>Directions:</u>

1. In a bowl, layer cooked rice as the base.

2. Top with shredded chicken, black beans, corn, lettuce, tomatoes, avocado, and cheese.

3. Drizzle with sour cream and salsa.

4. Garnish with lime wedges and fresh cilantro if desired.

5. Mix the ingredients together before eating.

<u>Nutrition Information (approx.):</u>

- Calories: 450-600

- Protein: 25-30g

- Carbohydrates: 50-60g

- Fat: 15-20g

- Fiber: 8-10g

22. Chicken Philly Croissant Loaf.

Ingredients:

- Cooked chicken slices

- Sliced bell peppers and onions

- Provolone or Swiss cheese slices

- Croissant loaf

- Mayonnaise

- Olive oil

- Salt and pepper

Directions:

1. Preheat oven to 350°F (175°C).

2. In a skillet, sauté bell peppers and onions in olive oil until tender.

3. Slice the croissant loaf lengthwise without separating the halves.

4. Spread mayonnaise on one side of the croissant loaf.

5. Layer cooked chicken, sautéed peppers, onions, and cheese slices.

6. Close the croissant loaf and wrap it in foil.

7. Bake for about 10-15 minutes until the cheese is melted and the croissant is warm.

Nutrition Information (approx.):

- Calories: 450-550
- Protein: 20-25g

- Carbohydrates: 30-40g

- Fat: 25-30g

- Fiber: 2-4g

23. Apple Yogurt Salad.

Ingredients:

- Mixed greens or spinach

- Sliced apples

- Greek yogurt

- Chopped nuts (such as walnuts or almonds)

- Dried cranberries or raisins

- Honey

- Lemon juice

Directions:

1. In a bowl, combine mixed greens, sliced apples, chopped nuts, and dried cranberries.
2. In a separate bowl, mix Greek yogurt with a drizzle of honey and a splash of lemon juice.
3. Toss the salad with the yogurt dressing just before serving.

Nutrition Information (approx.):

- Calories: 250-350
- Protein: 8-10g
- Carbohydrates: 30-40g
- Fat: 10-15g
- Fiber: 4-6g

24. Buffalo Chicken Wraps.

<u>*Ingredients:*</u>

- Cooked and shredded chicken (seasoned with buffalo sauce)
- Flour tortillas or wraps
- Shredded lettuce
- Chopped celery
- Blue cheese or ranch dressing
- Sliced red onion (optional)

<u>*Directions:*</u>

1. In a bowl, mix shredded chicken with buffalo sauce until coated.
2. Lay out tortillas and place shredded lettuce, chopped celery, and sliced red onion (if using) in the center.

3. Top with the buffalo chicken mixture.

4. Drizzle with blue cheese or ranch dressing.

5. Roll up the wraps tightly and secure with toothpicks if needed.

Nutrition Information (approx.):

- Calories: 350-450
- Protein: 25-30g
- Carbohydrates: 30-40g
- Fat: 15-20g
- Fiber: 3-5g

25. Spinach Cucumber Chicken and Ranch Wraps.

Ingredients:

- Cooked and sliced chicken breast
- Whole wheat tortillas or wraps
- Fresh spinach leaves
- Sliced cucumber
- Ranch dressing

Directions:

1. Lay out tortillas and place fresh spinach leaves on each.
2. Layer sliced chicken and sliced cucumber over the spinach.
3. Drizzle ranch dressing over the ingredients.
4. Roll up the wraps tightly and serve.

Nutrition Information (approx.):

- Calories: 300-400
- Protein: 20-25g
- Carbohydrates: 30-35g
- Fat: 12-15g
- Fiber: 5-7g

<u>Dinner Ideas</u> 🌑.

<u>26. Shrimp Foil Packet.</u>

<u>Ingredients:</u>

- 1 pound large shrimp, peeled and deveined
- 1 cup cherry tomatoes, halved
- 1 zucchini, sliced
- 1 yellow bell pepper, sliced
- 1 red onion, sliced
- 2 cloves garlic, minced
- 2 tablespoons olive oil
- 1 teaspoon dried oregano
- Salt and pepper to taste
- Fresh parsley, chopped (for garnish)

<u>*Directions:*</u>

1. Preheat your grill to medium-high heat.

2. In a large bowl, combine the shrimp, cherry tomatoes, zucchini, bell pepper, red onion, and minced garlic.

3. Drizzle the olive oil over the ingredients, then add the dried oregano, salt, and pepper. Toss to coat everything evenly.

4. Lay out a large piece of aluminum foil. Place the shrimp and vegetable mixture onto the foil.

5. Fold the foil over the ingredients and seal the edges to create a packet.

6. Place the foil packet on the preheated grill and cook for about 10-12 minutes, or until the shrimp are pink and opaque.

7. Carefully open the foil packet, garnish with chopped parsley, and serve.

Nutrition Information (per serving):

- Calories: ~250
- Protein: ~25g
- Carbohydrates: ~10g
- Fat: ~12g
- Fiber: ~2g

27. Crack Chicken Burgers

Ingredients:

- 1 pound ground chicken
- 1 packet ranch seasoning mix
- 8 slices cooked bacon

- 1 cup shredded cheddar cheese
- 4 hamburger buns
- Lettuce, tomato, and onion (for topping)

Directions:

1. In a mixing bowl, combine the ground chicken and ranch seasoning mix. Form into four burger patties.
2. Preheat a grill or stovetop skillet over medium-high heat.
3. Cook the chicken patties for about 5-6 minutes per side, or until fully cooked.
4. In the last minute of cooking, place a quarter of the shredded cheese on each patty to melt.
5. Assemble the burgers: Place each cooked patty on a bun, top with two slices of bacon, lettuce, tomato, and onion.

6. Serve with your favorite sides.

Nutrition Information (per serving):

- Calories: ~450
- Protein: ~35g
- Carbohydrates: ~25g
- Fat: ~25g
- Fiber: ~2g

28. Taco Fiesta Bubble Up Casserole.

Ingredients:

- 1 pound ground beef
- 1 packet taco seasoning

- 1 can (8 oz) refrigerated biscuit dough

- 1 cup salsa

- 1 cup shredded cheddar cheese

- 1 cup diced tomatoes

- 1/2 cup diced bell peppers

- 1/2 cup diced onions

- 1/2 cup sliced black olives

- 1/4 cup chopped fresh cilantro

Directions:

1. Preheat your oven to 375°F (190°C).

2. In a skillet, cook the ground beef over medium heat until browned. Drain excess fat.

3. Stir in the taco seasoning and cook according to the packet instructions.

4. Cut the biscuit dough into small pieces.

5. In a large bowl, combine the cooked beef, biscuit pieces, salsa, diced tomatoes, bell peppers, onions, and black olives.

6. Transfer the mixture to a greased 9x13-inch baking dish.

7. Top with shredded cheddar cheese.

8. Bake in the preheated oven for about 25-30 minutes, or until the biscuits are cooked through and the cheese is melted and bubbly.

9. Remove from the oven and sprinkle chopped cilantro on top.

10. Let it cool slightly before serving.

Nutrition Information (Approximate):

- Calories: 350 per serving
- Fat: 18g

- Carbohydrates: 27g

- Protein: 20g

29. Fettuccine in a Creamy Zucchini Sauce.

Ingredients:

- 8 oz fettuccine pasta

- 2 medium zucchinis, grated

- 2 cloves garlic, minced

- 1/4 cup heavy cream

- 1/4 cup grated Parmesan cheese

- 2 tablespoons butter

- Salt and pepper to taste

- Fresh basil leaves for garnish

Directions:

1. Cook the fettuccine pasta according to the package instructions. Drain and set aside.

2. In a large skillet, melt the butter over medium heat. Add the minced garlic and sauté for about 1 minute until fragrant.

3. Add the grated zucchinis to the skillet and cook for 3-4 minutes until they soften.

4. Stir in the heavy cream and grated Parmesan cheese.

5. Cook for an additional 2-3 minutes until the sauce thickens.

6. Season the sauce with salt and pepper to taste.

7. Toss the cooked fettuccine in the creamy zucchini sauce until well coated.

8. Serve the pasta in individual plates, garnished with fresh basil leaves.

__Nutrition Information (Approximate):__

- Calories: 400 per serving
- Fat: 18g
- Carbohydrates: 47g
- Protein: 12g

30. Chicken Parmesan Spaghetti Bake.

__Ingredients:__

- 8 oz spaghetti
- 2 cups cooked and diced chicken breast
- 2 cups marinara sauce
- 1 cup shredded mozzarella cheese
- 1/2 cup grated Parmesan cheese
- 1 teaspoon dried basil
- 1 teaspoon dried oregano

- 1/2 teaspoon garlic powder

- Salt and pepper to taste

- Fresh parsley for garnish

Directions:

1. Preheat your oven to 375°F (190°C).

2. Cook the spaghetti according to the package instructions. Drain and set aside.

3. In a large bowl, combine the cooked diced chicken, marinara sauce, dried basil, dried oregano, garlic powder, salt, and pepper.

4. In a greased 9x13-inch baking dish, spread half of the cooked spaghetti.

5. Top the spaghetti with half of the chicken and sauce mixture.

6. Sprinkle half of the shredded mozzarella and grated Parmesan cheese over the chicken layer.

7. Repeat the layers with the remaining spaghetti, chicken and sauce mixture, and cheeses.

8. Bake in the preheated oven for about 20-25 minutes, until the cheese is melted and bubbly.

9. Garnish with fresh parsley before serving.

Nutrition Information (Approximate):

- Calories: 420 per serving
- Fat: 14g
- Carbohydrates: 44g
- Protein: 30g

Soups

31. Slow Cooker Beef and Barley Soup.

Ingredients:

- 1 lb beef stew meat, cubed
- 1 cup pearl barley
- 3 carrots, peeled and chopped
- 2 celery stalks, chopped
- 1 onion, chopped
- 3 cloves garlic, minced
- 6 cups beef broth
- 1 can diced tomatoes
- 2 tsp dried thyme
- Salt and pepper to taste

<u>*Directions:*</u>

1. In a skillet, brown the beef cubes on all sides. Transfer to the slow cooker.
2. Add the chopped carrots, celery, onion, and garlic to the slow cooker.
3. Pour in the beef broth and diced tomatoes.
4. Stir in the pearl barley and dried thyme. Add salt and pepper to taste.
5. Cover and cook on low for 6-8 hours or until the beef and barley are tender.
6. Adjust seasoning if needed before serving.

<u>*Nutrition Information:*</u>

- (Per serving, about 1.5 cups)
- Calories: 250
- Protein: 18g
- Carbohydrates: 28g

- Fat: 6g
- Fiber: 5g

32. Buffalo Chicken Soup

Ingredients:

- 2 boneless, skinless chicken breasts
- 4 cups chicken broth
- 1 cup chopped celery
- 1 cup chopped carrots
- 1 onion, diced
- 2 cloves garlic, minced
- 1/2 cup hot sauce (adjust to taste)
- 1 cup heavy cream
- 1 cup shredded cheddar cheese
- Salt and pepper to taste

Directions:

1. Place chicken breasts, chicken broth, celery, carrots, onion, and garlic in the slow cooker.
2. Cook on low for 6-8 hours or until the chicken is cooked through and vegetables are tender.
3. Remove the chicken, shred it, and return to the slow cooker.
4. Stir in hot sauce and heavy cream. Add salt and pepper to taste.
5. Before serving, stir in shredded cheddar cheese until melted.

Nutrition Information:

- (Per serving, about 1.5 cups)
- Calories: 350

- Protein: 25g

- Carbohydrates: 10g

- Fat: 24g

- Fiber: 2g

33. Chicken Taco Soup.

Ingredients:

- 2 boneless, skinless chicken breasts

- 1 can black beans, drained and rinsed

- 1 can corn, drained

- 1 can diced tomatoes with green chilies

- 1 onion, diced

- 2 cloves garlic, minced

- 1 packet taco seasoning

- 4 cups chicken broth

- Optional toppings: shredded cheese, sour cream, tortilla strips

Directions:

1. Place chicken breasts, black beans, corn, diced tomatoes, onion, and garlic in the slow cooker.
2. Sprinkle taco seasoning over the ingredients.
3. Pour in the chicken broth.
4. Cook on low for 6-8 hours or until the chicken is cooked through and flavors are well blended.
5. Remove the chicken, shred it, and return to the soup.
6. Serve with optional toppings, if desired.

Nutrition Information:

- (Per serving, about 1.5 cups)

- Calories: 280

- Protein: 20g

- Carbohydrates: 32g

- Fat: 6g

- Fiber: 7g

34. Slow Cooker Cabbage Roll Soup.

Ingredients:

- 1 lb ground beef

- 1 onion, chopped

- 2 cloves garlic, minced

- 4 cups beef broth

- 1 can diced tomatoes

- 1 cup tomato sauce

- 1 cup chopped cabbage

- 1/2 cup chopped carrots

- 1/2 cup chopped celery

- 1/2 cup rice

- 1 tsp dried thyme

- Salt and pepper to taste

Directions:

1. In a skillet, brown the ground beef along with onion and garlic. Drain excess fat.

2. Transfer the beef mixture to the slow cooker.

3. Add beef broth, diced tomatoes, tomato sauce, chopped cabbage, carrots, celery, rice, dried thyme, salt, and pepper.

4. Stir well and cook on low for 6-8 hours or until the rice and vegetables are tender.

5. Adjust seasoning if needed before serving.

Nutrition Information:

- (Per serving, about 1.5 cups)
- Calories: 320
- Protein: 18g
- Carbohydrates: 32g
- Fat: 13g
- Fiber: 4g

35. Chicken Noodle Soup

Ingredients:

- 2 boneless, skinless chicken breasts
- 4 cups chicken broth
- 4 cups water
- 2 carrots, peeled and sliced

- 2 celery stalks, sliced

- 1 onion, chopped

- 2 cloves garlic, minced

- 2 cups egg noodles

- 1 tsp dried thyme

- Salt and pepper to taste

- Fresh parsley for garnish

Directions:

1. Place chicken breasts, chicken broth, water, carrots, celery, onion, and garlic in the slow cooker.

2. Cook on low for 6-8 hours or until the chicken is cooked through and vegetables are tender.

3. Remove the chicken, shred it, and return to the soup.

4. Stir in egg noodles and dried thyme.

5. Cook on low for an additional 20-30 minutes or until noodles are tender.

6. Season with salt and pepper.

7. Garnish with fresh parsley before serving.

Nutrition Information:

- (Per serving, about 1.5 cups)
- Calories: 280
- Protein: 20g
- Carbohydrates: 30g
- Fat: 7g
- Fiber: 3g

Snacks

36. Turkey Sausage Rolls.

Ingredients:

- 1 pound ground turkey sausage
- 1 sheet puff pastry, thawed
- 1 egg, beaten (for egg wash)
- 1 teaspoon dried sage
- 1/2 teaspoon dried thyme
- Salt and pepper to taste

Directions:

1. Preheat the oven to 375°F (190°C) and line a baking sheet with parchment paper.

2. In a bowl, combine the ground turkey sausage, dried sage, dried thyme, salt, and pepper. Mix well.

3. Roll out the puff pastry sheet on a floured surface. Cut it into smaller squares.

4. Place a spoonful of the turkey sausage mixture onto each pastry square. Fold the pastry over the filling and press the edges to seal. Repeat for all squares.

5. Brush the tops of the rolls with beaten egg to give them a golden color when baked.

6. Place the rolls on the prepared baking sheet and bake for about 20-25 minutes, or until the pastry is golden brown and the sausage is cooked through.

Nutrition Information:

- Calories: 250 per roll

- Protein: 10g per roll

- Carbohydrates: 15g per roll

- Fat: 16g per roll

37. Onion Cheese Rings.

Ingredients:

- 2 large onions, sliced into rings

- 1 cup all-purpose flour

- 1 teaspoon paprika

- 1/2 teaspoon garlic powder

- Salt and pepper to taste

- 1 cup buttermilk

- 1 cup bread crumbs

- 1 cup shredded cheddar cheese

- Cooking oil for frying

<u>*Directions:*</u>

1. In a bowl, mix the flour, paprika, garlic powder, salt, and pepper.
2. Dip each onion ring into the flour mixture, shaking off any excess.
3. Dip the floured onion rings into the buttermilk, allowing any excess to drip off.
4. Coat the onion rings with bread crumbs mixed with shredded cheddar cheese.
5. Heat oil in a deep fryer or heavy skillet to 350°F (175°C).
6. Fry the coated onion rings in batches until they are golden brown and crispy. Remove and place on paper towels to drain excess oil.

- Calories: 180 per serving (6-8 rings)
- Protein: 7g per serving
- Carbohydrates: 20g per serving
- Fat: 8g per serving

38. Pumpkin Spice Granola.

<u>*Ingredients:*</u>

- 3 cups old-fashioned oats
- 1 cup pumpkin puree
- 1/2 cup honey or maple syrup
- 1/2 cup chopped nuts (e.g., pecans, almonds)
- 1/2 cup dried cranberries or raisins

- 1 teaspoon pumpkin pie spice

- 1/2 teaspoon vanilla extract

- Pinch of salt

Directions:

1. Preheat the oven to 325°F (165°C) and line a baking sheet with parchment paper.

2. In a bowl, mix together the pumpkin puree, honey or maple syrup, pumpkin pie spice, vanilla extract, and a pinch of salt.

3. Add the oats and chopped nuts to the wet mixture, stirring until everything is well combined.

4. Spread the mixture evenly onto the prepared baking sheet.

5. Bake for about 20-25 minutes, stirring halfway through, until the granola is golden and crisp.

6. Remove from the oven and let the granola cool completely. Once cooled, mix in the dried cranberries or raisins.

Nutrition Information:

- Calories: 180 per 1/2 cup serving
- Protein: 4g per serving
- Carbohydrates: 30g per serving
- Fat: 5g per serving

39. Garlic Cheddar Biscuits.

Ingredients:

- 2 cups all-purpose flour
- 1 tablespoon baking powder

- 1/2 teaspoon salt

- 1/2 teaspoon garlic powder

- 1/2 cup cold unsalted butter, cubed

- 1 cup shredded cheddar cheese

- 3/4 cup milk

- 2 tablespoons chopped fresh parsley

- 2 tablespoons melted butter

- 1/2 teaspoon garlic powder

Directions:

1. Preheat the oven to 425°F (220°C) and line a baking sheet with parchment paper.

2. In a bowl, whisk together the flour, baking powder, salt, and garlic powder.

3. Cut in the cold butter using a pastry cutter or your fingers until the mixture resembles coarse crumbs.

4. Stir in the shredded cheddar cheese.

5. Gradually add the milk and mix until just combined.

6. Drop spoonfuls of the dough onto the prepared baking sheet to make biscuits.

7. Bake for about 12-15 minutes, or until the biscuits are golden brown.

8. In a small bowl, mix melted butter and garlic powder. Brush this mixture over the freshly baked biscuits and sprinkle with chopped parsley.

Nutrition Information:

- Calories: 220 per biscuit
- Protein: 5g per biscuit
- Carbohydrates: 20g per biscuit
- Fat: 13g per biscuit

Dessert.

40. Blueberry Lemon Cannolis.

Ingredients:

- 8 cannoli shells
- 1 cup ricotta cheese
- 1/2 cup powdered sugar
- 1/2 teaspoon vanilla extract
- Zest of 1 lemon
- 1/2 cup fresh blueberries

Directions:

1. In a mixing bowl, combine the ricotta cheese, powdered sugar, vanilla extract, and lemon zest. Mix until smooth.

2. Gently fold in the fresh blueberries.

3. Fill the cannoli shells with the ricotta mixture using a pastry bag or a spoon.

4. Refrigerate for at least 30 minutes before serving to allow flavors to meld.

5. Optional: Dust with powdered sugar and garnish with additional lemon zest before serving.

Nutrition Information (per cannoli):

- Calories: Approximately 180
- Protein: 4g
- Carbohydrates: 20g
- Fat: 10g
- Fiber: 1g

- Sugars: 10g

41. Mini Mint Oreo Cheesecake Bites.

Ingredients:

- 12 Oreo cookies
- 8 oz cream cheese, softened
- 1/4 cup granulated sugar
- 1 egg
- 1/2 teaspoon peppermint extract
- Green food coloring (optional)
- Whipped cream and mini Oreo cookies for garnish

Directions:

1. Preheat the oven to 325°F (165°C) and line a mini muffin tin with paper liners.

2. Place one Oreo cookie at the bottom of each liner.

3. In a mixing bowl, beat the cream cheese and granulated sugar until smooth.

4. Add the egg, peppermint extract, and green food coloring (if using), and mix until well combined.

5. Spoon the cream cheese mixture over the Oreo cookies in the liners, filling each almost to the top.

6. Bake for about 15-18 minutes, until the cheesecakes are set but slightly jiggly in the center.

7. Let the cheesecakes cool in the muffin tin, then refrigerate for at least 2 hours or until fully chilled.

8. Garnish with whipped cream and mini Oreo cookies before serving.

Nutrition Information (per cheesecake bite):

- Calories: Approximately 150
- Protein: 2g
- Carbohydrates: 13g
- Fat: 10g
- Sugar: 10g
-

42. Apple Strudels.

Ingredients:

- 2 medium apples, peeled, cored, and thinly sliced

- 1/4 cup granulated sugar

- 1 teaspoon ground cinnamon

- 1/4 cup breadcrumbs

- 1/4 cup chopped walnuts or almonds

- 4 sheets phyllo dough

- 1/4 cup unsalted butter, melted

- Powdered sugar for dusting

Directions:

1. Preheat the oven to 375°F (190°C).

2. In a bowl, combine the sliced apples, granulated sugar, and ground cinnamon.

3. Let it sit for a few minutes to release the juices.

4. Mix in the breadcrumbs and chopped nuts to the apple mixture.

5. Lay out one sheet of phyllo dough and brush it with melted butter. Repeat with 3

more sheets, stacking them on top of each other.

6. Spread the apple filling along one edge of the phyllo stack.

7. Roll the phyllo dough tightly, enclosing the apple filling, to create a strudel shape.

8. Place the strudel on a baking sheet lined with parchment paper, seam side down. Brush the top with more melted butter.

9. Bake for about 25-30 minutes, until the strudel is golden brown and crispy.

10. Let the strudel cool slightly before dusting with powdered sugar.

Nutrition Information (per serving):

- Calories: Approximately 250
- Protein: 3g
- Carbohydrates: 31g

- Fat: 13g
- Fiber: 3g
- Sugars: 15g

International Flavors.

43. Vegetable Upma (Indian Semolina Breakfast).

Ingredients:

- 1 cup semolina (rava)
- 1/4 cup chopped mixed vegetables (carrots, peas, bell peppers)
- 2 tablespoons oil or ghee
- 1 teaspoon mustard seeds
- 1 teaspoon cumin seeds
- 1/2 teaspoon urad dal (split black gram)
- 1/2 teaspoon chana dal (split chickpeas)

- 1/4 teaspoon asafoetida (hing)
- 1 green chili, chopped
- 1 teaspoon grated ginger
- Curry leaves
- Cashew nuts (optional)
- Salt, to taste
- Water, as needed

Directions:

1. Heat oil in a pan, add mustard seeds and let them splutter. Add cumin seeds, urad dal, and chana dal. Sauté until dals turn golden.
2. Add cashew nuts (if using), grcen chili, grated ginger, and curry leaves. Sauté for a minute.

3. Add chopped vegetables and sauté until they are slightly cooked.

4. In another pan, dry roast semolina until it turns aromatic and slightly changes color.

5. Add roasted semolina to the pan with vegetables. Mix well.

6. Add water (typically in a 1:2 ratio of semolina to water) and salt. Stir continuously to prevent lumps. Cook until the mixture thickens and semolina is cooked.

7. Serve hot garnished with chopped cilantro.

Nutrition Information (approximate, per serving):

- Calories: 220 kcal
- Carbohydrates: 40g

- Protein: 5g

- Fat: 5g

- Fiber: 3g

44. Japanese Tamago Sando (Egg Salad Sandwich).

Ingredients:

- 4 large eggs

- 2 tablespoons mayonnaise

- 1 teaspoon soy sauce

- Salt and pepper, to taste

- 8 slices of bread (white or milk bread works well)

- Butter, for spreading

- Optional: thinly sliced cucumber or lettuce for extra crunch

<u>Directions:</u>

1. Place the eggs in a saucepan and cover them with water.

2. Bring the water to a boil, then reduce the heat to a gentle simmer. Cook the eggs for about 9-10 minutes.

3. While the eggs are cooking, prepare a bowl of ice water. Once the eggs are done cooking, transfer them immediately to the ice water to cool. This helps in easy peeling and prevents overcooking.

4. Once the eggs are completely cooled, peel them and chop them finely.

5. In a bowl, mix the chopped eggs, mayonnaise, soy sauce, salt, and pepper.

6. Adjust the seasoning to your taste.

7. Butter one side of each slice of bread.

8. Place a generous amount of the egg salad mixture on the unbuttered side of half of the slices.

9. If you're using cucumber or lettuce, layer a few slices on top of the egg salad.

10. Top with the remaining slices of bread, buttered side facing out.

11. Optionally, trim the crusts from the sandwiches for a more authentic look. Then, cut the sandwiches into halves or quarters.

12. Your Japanese Tamago Sando is ready to be enjoyed!

13. Serve them as is, or wrap them in plastic wrap for a convenient on-the-go meal.

Nutrition Information.

- Calories: 250 kcal

- Carbohydrates: 25g

- Protein: 12g

- Fat: 11g

- Fiber: 2g

45..Mexican Breakfast Tacos with Black Beans

Ingredients:

- 4 small flour or corn tortillas

- 1 cup cooked black beans

- 4 large eggs

- Salt and black pepper, to taste

- 1/2 cup diced tomatoes

- 1/4 cup diced red onion

- 1/4 cup chopped fresh cilantro
- Salsa or hot sauce, for serving
- Lime wedges, for serving

Directions:

1. Heat the tortillas in a dry skillet or oven until warm.
2. In a pan, heat the cooked black beans. Season with salt and black pepper.
3. In another pan, scramble the eggs. Season with salt and black pepper.
4. To assemble the tacos, place a spoonful of black beans on each tortilla.
5. Top with scrambled eggs, diced tomatoes, diced red onion, and chopped cilantro.
6. Serve with salsa or hot sauce on the side and lime wedges for squeezing.

<u>*Nutrition Information .*</u>

- Calories: 230 kcal
- Carbohydrates: 28g
- Protein: 11g
- Fat: 8g
- Fiber: 7g